KNOWLEDGE ON BREAST CANCER

(All you need to know to win breast cancer)

MILDRED .G. BARBEAU

TABLE OF CONTENTS

PREFACE

Breast cancer is a topic that affects millions of people around the world, and its impact on individuals and families can be profound. As a medical professional and breast cancer researcher, I have seen firsthand the devastating effects that this disease can have on patients and their loved ones.

It is my hope that this book, "Knowledge on Breast Cancer," will serve as a comprehensive guide to understanding the disease and navigating its diagnosis and treatment. Whether you are a patient, caregiver, or simply seeking to educate yourself on breast cancer, this book is intended to provide the essential knowledge and guidance you need.

Throughout the pages of this book, you will find a wealth of information on the science behind breast cancer, including its causes, risk factors, and diagnosis. You will also learn about the latest advances in cancer treatment, including innovative new therapies and surgical techniques.

But this book is more than just a clinical guide to breast cancer. It is also a resource for understanding the emotional and psychological impact of the disease, and for finding the support and resources you need to navigate this challenging journey.

Ultimately, my goal in writing this book is to empower individuals and families affected by breast cancer with the knowledge and tools they need to make informed decisions about their care and to find hope and healing in the face of this difficult diagnosis.

BREASTS OVERVIEW

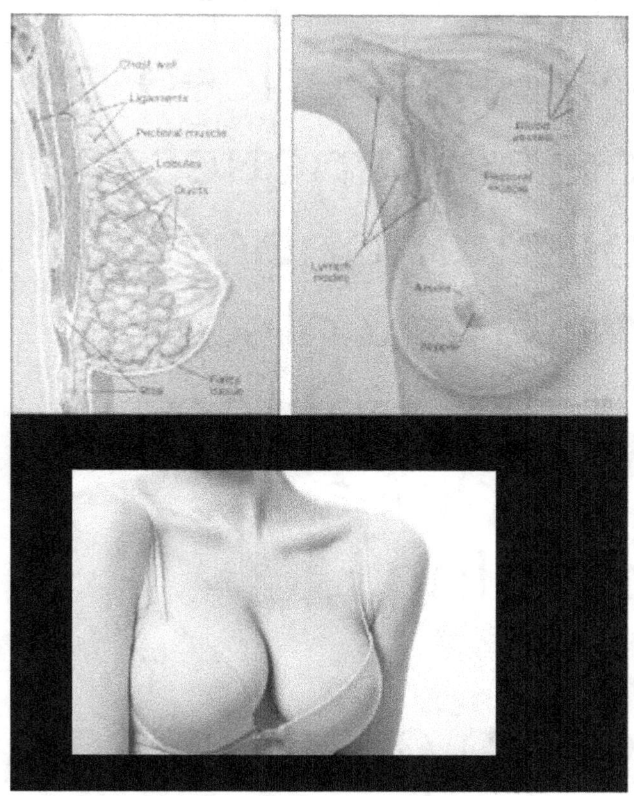

Breasts, also known as **mammary glands,** are an essential part of the female reproductive system. They are located on the chest wall of females and consist of glandular and fatty tissue. Breasts are responsible for producing and secreting milk for newborn infants during breastfeeding.

Breasts come in various shapes and sizes and can be influenced by several factors such as genetics, age, weight, hormonal changes, and pregnancy. They may also change over time due to factors such as weight gain or loss, breastfeeding, and aging.

While breasts are often associated with femininity and beauty, they also have a significant impact on a woman's health. Regular breast self-examinations, clinical breast exams, and mammograms are essential for detecting and treating breast cancer, which is the most common cancer among women worldwide.

Overall, breasts play an important role in both reproduction and overall health, and it is essential to take care of them through proper breast health practices and regular medical check-ups.

EVOLUTION OF BREAST CANCER

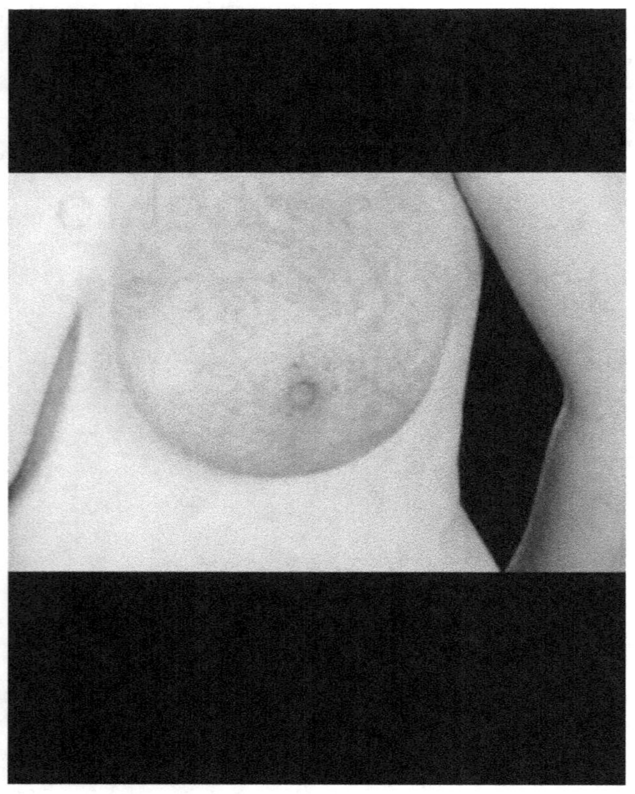

Breast cancer is a disease that has evolved over time, both in terms of our understanding of the disease and its treatment options. Here are some key milestones in the evolution of breast cancer:

- **Early history**: Breast cancer has been recognized as a disease since ancient times. The Edwin Smith Papyrus, an ancient Egyptian medical text dating back to 1600 BC, describes cases of breast cancer and recommends surgical removal of the tumor.

- **19th century**: The first modern surgical techniques for breast cancer, including radical mastectomy, were developed in the 19th century. However, these surgeries were often disfiguring and associated with high rates of morbidity and mortality.

- **20th century**: In the early 20th century, radiation therapy was introduced as a treatment option for breast cancer. Chemotherapy was also developed in the mid-20th century and became a mainstay of breast cancer treatment in the following decades.

- **Late 20th century**: In the 1980s and 1990s, advances in breast cancer research led to the identification of specific genetic mutations.

WHAT CAUSES BREAST CANCER?

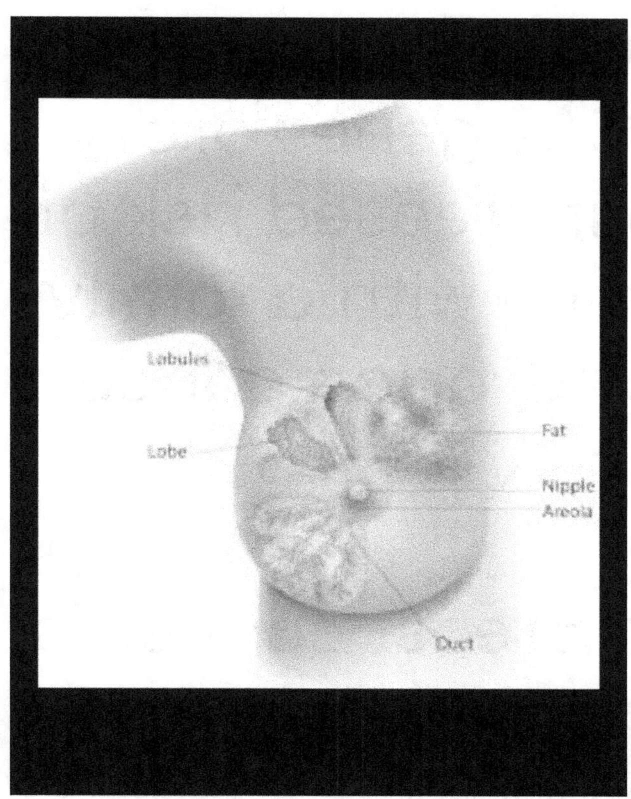

Breast cancer occurs when cells in the breast start to grow uncontrollably, forming a tumor. While the exact cause of breast cancer is not fully understood, there are several risk factors that can increase the likelihood of developing the disease:

1. **Genetics**: Inherited mutations in the **BRCA1** and **BRCA2** genes are responsible for an increased risk of breast cancer. Women with a family history of breast or ovarian cancer are also at higher risk.

2. **Age and gender**: Breast cancer is more common in women, and the risk increases with age.

3. **Hormones**: Exposure to estrogen and progesterone, particularly in women who have had a prolonged exposure, such as early onset of menstruation, late onset of menopause, or use of hormonal contraceptives, can increase the risk.

4. **Lifestyle factors**: Obesity, lack of physical activity, and alcohol consumption have been linked to an increased risk of breast cancer.

5. **Radiation exposure**: Exposure to radiation, particularly during adolescence or early adulthood, can increase the risk of developing breast cancer later in life.

It is important to note that having one or more of these risk factors does not necessarily mean a person will develop breast cancer, and many people with breast cancer have no identifiable risk factors. Early detection through regular breast cancer screening is crucial for successful treatment and recovery.

STAGES OF BREAST CANCER.

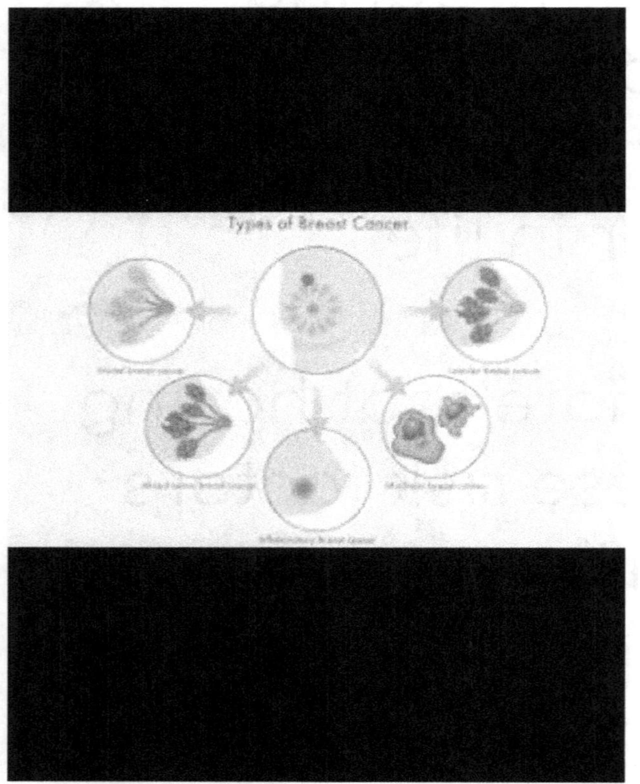

Breast cancer is classified into different stages based on the size and extent of the tumor and whether it has spread to nearby lymph nodes or other parts of the body. The most commonly used staging system is the TNM system, which stands for tumor, nodes, and metastasis. Here are the stages of breast cancer according to the TNM system:

Stage 0 (DCIS): Ductal carcinoma in situ (DCIS) is a non-invasive breast cancer that is confined to the milk ducts of the breast and has not spread to nearby tissue.

Stage I: In stage I, the tumor is small and has not spread beyond the breast tissue. The cancer has not spread to nearby lymph nodes.

Stage II: In stage II, the tumor is larger or has spread to nearby lymph nodes, but has not yet spread to other parts of the body.

Stage III: In stage III, the tumor has spread to nearby lymph nodes and may have spread to surrounding tissues, such as the chest wall or skin.

Stage IV: In stage IV, the cancer has spread to other parts of the body, such as the lungs, liver, or bones. This is also known as **metastatic breast cancer.**

Within each stage, there may be sub-stages that further describe the extent of the cancer. The stage of breast cancer is an important factor in determining the most appropriate treatment options and predicting the prognosis for the patient.

LIFESTYLE THAT ENHANCES BREAST CANCER

There are several lifestyle factors that may increase a person's risk of developing breast cancer, including:

1. **Lack Of Physical Activity:** Being physically inactive can increase the risk of breast cancer.

2. **Obesity**: Being overweight or obese, particularly after menopause, can increase the risk of breast cancer.

3. **Alcohol consumption**: Consuming alcohol, particularly more than one drink per day, can increase the risk of breast cancer.

4. **Hormonal contraceptives**: Some hormonal contraceptives, such as birth control pills or hormone-releasing intrauterine devices **(IUDs)**, may increase the risk of breast cancer.

5. **Hormone therapy**: Hormone replacement therapy **(HRT)** for menopause, particularly when

taken for a long time, can increase the risk of breast cancer.

6. **Smoking**: Smoking has been linked to an increased risk of breast cancer, particularly in younger women.

7. **Diet**: A diet high in saturated fat and low in fruits and vegetables may increase the risk of breast cancer.

It is important to note that having one or more of these risk factors does not necessarily mean a person will develop breast cancer, and many people with breast cancer have no identifiable risk factors. However, adopting a healthy lifestyle can reduce the risk of many diseases, including breast cancer.

FOODS THAT CAN HEIGHTEN THE RISK OF BREAST CANCER

While there is no specific food or diet that is known to cause breast cancer, there are certain foods that may increase a person's risk of developing the disease. Here are some examples:

1. **High-fat diets**: Diets high in saturated and trans fats, found in red meat, fried foods, and processed snacks, have been linked to an increased risk of breast cancer.

2. **Excessive alcohol consumption:**
Consuming alcohol, particularly
more than one drink per day, has
been linked to an increased risk of
breast cancer.

3. **Processed and packaged foods:**
Processed and packaged foods
may contain preservatives,
additives, and chemicals that can
contribute to the development of
breast cancer.

4. **Sugary foods and drinks:**
Consuming foods and drinks high
in added sugars, such as soda,
candy, and baked goods, can lead
to weight gain and increase the risk
of breast cancer.

5. **Soy products**: While soy products contain phytoestrogens, which may have protective effects against breast cancer, consuming large amounts of soy products may increase the risk of breast cancer in some women.

It is important to note that eating a healthy and balanced diet, rich in fruits, vegetables, whole grains, and lean proteins, can help reduce the risk of many diseases, including breast cancer. Additionally, maintaining a healthy weight, exercising regularly, and limiting alcohol consumption can also help lower the risk of breast cancer.

SYMPTOMS OF BREAST CANCER

Breast cancer may not always cause symptoms in its early stages, which is why it is important to undergo regular screenings. However, some common symptoms of breast cancer include:

1. **A lump or thickening in the breast or armpit:** A new lump or mass in the breast or underarm can be a sign of breast cancer. However, not all lumps are cancerous.

2. **Changes in breast size, shape, or appearance:** Breast cancer can cause changes in the size, shape, or appearance of the breast, such

as swelling, dimpling, or puckering of the skin.

3. **Nipple changes**: Changes in the nipple, such as inversion, redness, or discharge, can be a sign of breast cancer.

4. **Breast pain or tenderness**: While breast pain is usually not a symptom of breast cancer, it can be a sign of other breast conditions.

5. **Skin changes**: Changes in the skin over the breast, such as redness, scaling, or flakiness, can be a sign of breast cancer.

It is important to note that these symptoms may also be caused by other conditions, and having one or more of these symptoms does not necessarily mean a person has breast cancer. However, if a person notices any changes in their breasts, they should consult a healthcare provider for evaluation.

CHEMOTHERAPY

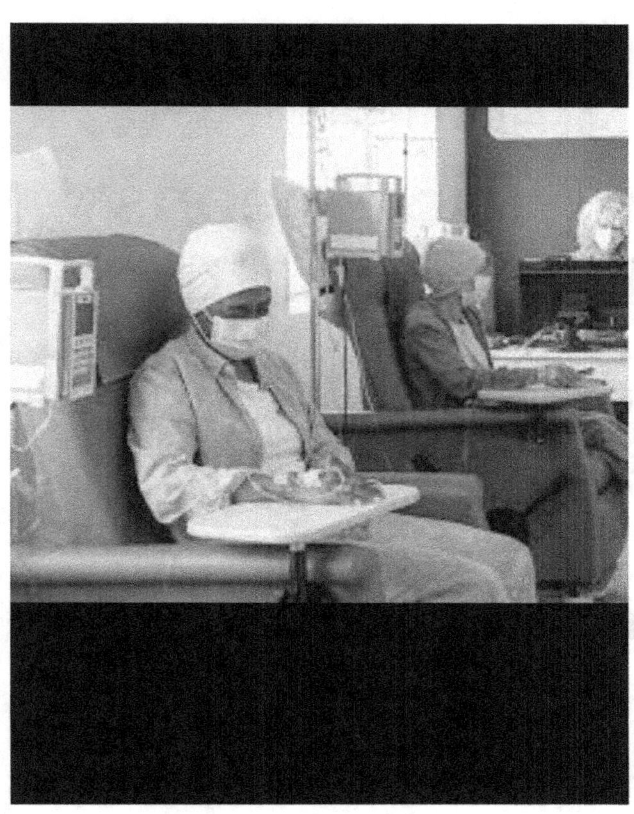

Chemotherapy is a type of cancer treatment that uses drugs to kill cancer cells. These drugs are usually administered intravenously, but can also be given orally or injected into a muscle or under the skin. Chemotherapy drugs work by targeting rapidly dividing cells, such as cancer cells, and stopping them from dividing and growing.

Chemotherapy is often used as a systemic treatment, which means that it circulates throughout the body to treat cancer cells wherever they may be. Depending on the type and stage of cancer, chemotherapy may be used alone or in combination with other treatments, such as surgery or radiation therapy.

Chemotherapy is associated with various side effects, as it can also affect normal cells that divide rapidly, such as those in the hair follicles and digestive tract. Common side effects include nausea, vomiting, hair loss, fatigue, and an increased risk of infections. These side effects can usually be managed with medications and lifestyle adjustments, and they tend to improve after treatment is completed.

The type, dose, and duration of chemotherapy depend on several factors, such as the type and stage of cancer, the person's overall health, and their response to treatment. A healthcare provider will work with the person to determine the most appropriate chemotherapy regimen for their specific situation.

Foods that help to prevent breast cancer
While there is no one food or diet that can completely prevent breast cancer, there are several foods that have been linked to a lower risk of developing the disease. Here are some examples:

1. **Fruits and vegetables**: Eating a variety of fruits and vegetables, particularly those that are brightly

colored and rich in antioxidants, can help reduce the risk of breast cancer.

2. **Whole grains**: Eating whole grains, such as brown rice, quinoa, and whole wheat bread, can help reduce the risk of breast cancer.

3. **Lean proteins**: Consuming lean proteins, such as fish, chicken, and legumes, can help maintain a healthy weight and reduce the risk of breast cancer.

4. **Nuts and seeds**: Eating nuts and seeds, such as almonds, walnuts, and flaxseed, can help reduce the risk of breast cancer due to their

high content of healthy fats and
fiber.

5. **Cruciferous vegetables:**
Vegetables in the cruciferous family,
such as broccoli, kale, and
cauliflower, contain compounds
that may help reduce the risk of
breast cancer.

6. **Green tea:** Drinking green tea,
which contains antioxidants called
catechins, may help reduce the risk
of breast cancer.

It is important to note that eating a
healthy and balanced diet is just
one of many lifestyle factors that
can help reduce the risk of breast
cancer. Other factors, such as

maintaining a healthy weight, exercising regularly, limiting alcohol consumption, and avoiding tobacco products, can also play a role in preventing breast cancer.

PREVENTIVE MEASURES OF BREAST CANC.

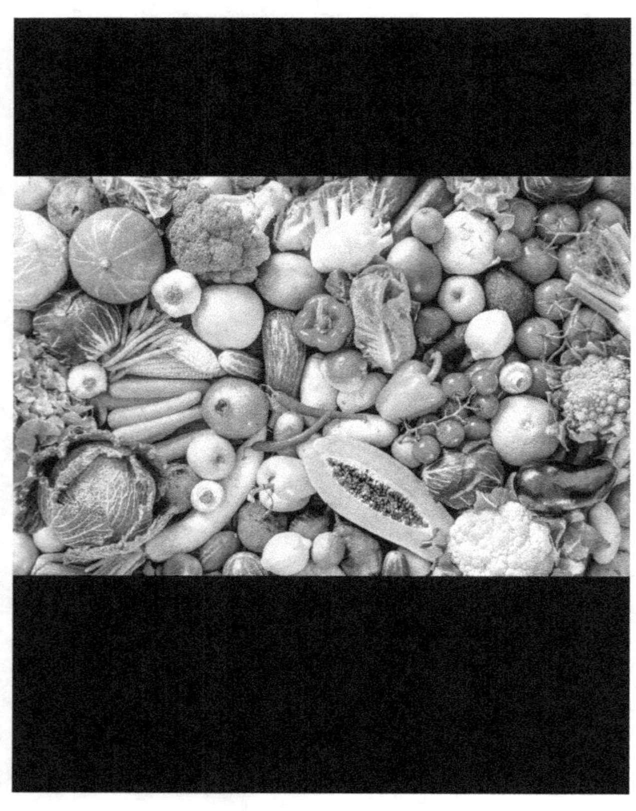

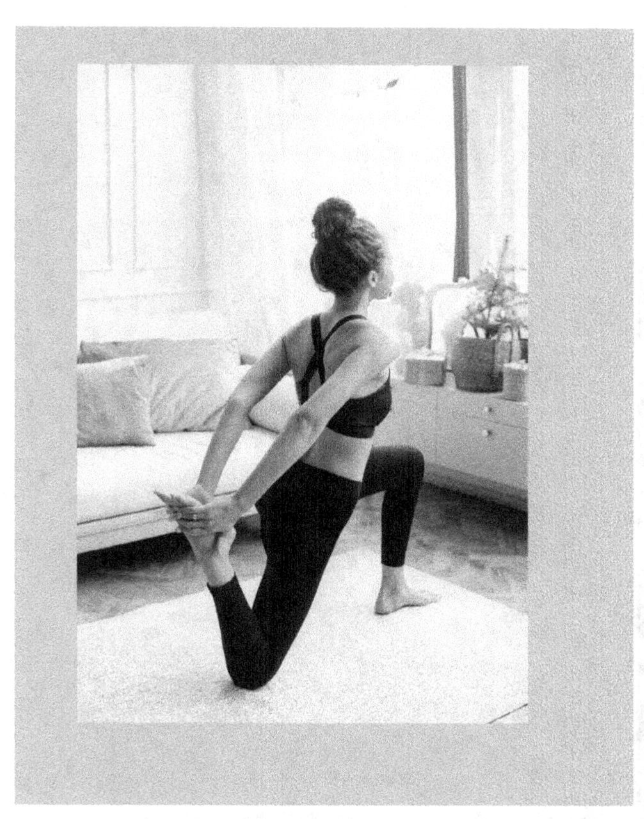

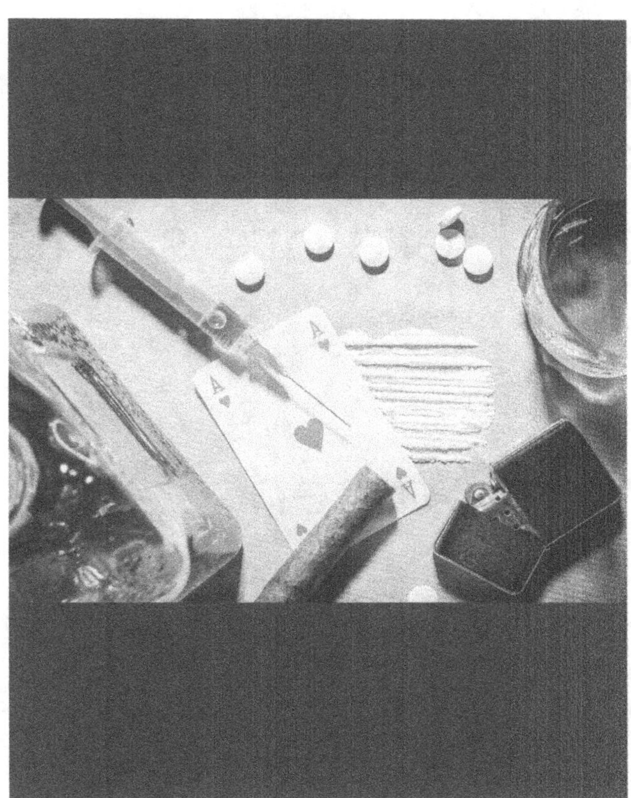

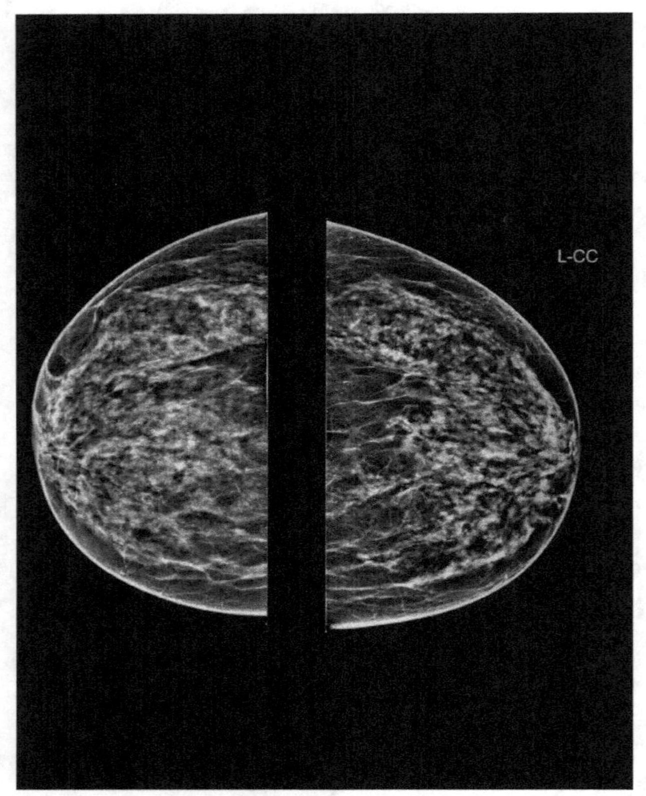

There are several preventive measures that can help reduce the risk of breast cancer. Here are some examples:

1. **Regular screenings**: Women should undergo regular screenings for breast cancer, such as mammograms, to detect any

abnormalities in the breast tissue early on.

2. **Maintain a healthy weight:** Being overweight or obese can increase the risk of breast cancer, so maintaining a healthy weight through a balanced diet and regular exercise is important.

3. **Limit alcohol consumption:** Consuming alcohol in excess can increase the risk of breast cancer, so it is recommended to limit alcohol consumption to no more than one drink per day.

4. **Breastfeeding:** Women who breastfeed their babies for at least

six months may have a lower risk of developing breast cancer.

5. **Avoid tobacco products**: Smoking and other tobacco products have been linked to an increased risk of breast cancer, so avoiding these products is important.

6. **Hormone therapy**: Women who undergo hormone therapy, such as estrogen and progesterone therapy, to treat menopause symptoms may have a higher risk of developing breast cancer. It is important to discuss the risks and benefits of hormone therapy with a healthcare provider.

7. **Genetic testing**: Women with a family history of breast cancer may benefit from genetic testing to determine if they carry certain gene mutations that increase the risk of breast cancer.

It is important to note that no single factor can completely prevent breast cancer, but by adopting a healthy lifestyle and discussing risk factors with a healthcare provider, women can take steps to reduce their risk of developing the disease.